Multiple-choice Q
Upper Diges

Other Examination Preparation Books Published by Petroc Press:

Balcombe	*Notes for the MRCP Part I*	190060342X
Bateson	*Basic Tests in Gastroenterology*	1900603772
Bateson	*MCQs in Clinical Gastroenterology*	1900603519
Bateson	*MCQs on the Upper Digestive Tract*	1900603373
Bateson & Stephen	*MCQs in Gastroenterology*	1900603403
Black & Kelleher	*MCQs in Anaesthesiology*	1900603454
Chakravorty	*Visual Aids to the MRCP Examination*	0792388739
Chong & Wong	*Survival Kit for MRCP Part II*	1900603063
Edgell	*Preparing for MRCP Part II Cardiology*	0792388690
Green	*More MCQs for Finals*	079238928X
Green (Ed.)	*The MRCPsych Study Manual:* 2nd edn	1900603527
Helmy & Mokbel	*Preparing for the PLAB Part 1*	1900603721
Hogston	*MCQs for the MRCoG Part II*	1900603551
Kubba *et al.*	*MCQs for MFFP Part I*	1900603004
Levi	*Basic Notes in Psychiatry:* 2nd edn	1900603306
Levi	*Basic Notes in Psychotherapy*	1900603500
Levi	*Basic Notes in Psychopharmacology:* 2nd edn	1900603608
Levi	*MCQs in Psychiatry for MRCPsych*	1900603853
Levi	*PMPs for the MRCPsych Part II*	079238993X
Levi	*SAQs for the MRCPsych*	0746200994
Levy & Riordan Eva	*MCQs in Optics and Refraction*	1900603225
Levy & Riordan Eva	*MCQs for the FRCOphth*	1900603276
Levy & Riordan Eva	*MCQs for the MRCOphth*	1900603179
Mokbel	*MCQs in Applied Basic Medical Sciences*	1900603756
Mokbel	*MCQs in General Surgery*	1900603101
Mokbel	*MCQs in Neurology*	0792388577
Mokbel *et al.*	*MCQs for the MRCP Part I*	1900603071
Mokbel	*Operative Surgery and Surgical Topics for the FRCS/MRCS*	1900603705
Mokbel	*SAQs in Clinical Surgery-in-General for the FRCS*	190060390X
Ross & Emmanuel	*MCQs on Antimicrobial Therapy*	1900603411
Ross & Emmanuel	*MCQs in Medical Microbiology for MRCP*	0792388836
Ross & Emmanuel	*MCQs in Medical Microbiology and Infectious Diseases*	1900603365
Ross & Emmanuel	*MCQs in Microbiology and Infection for FRCS*	1900603152
Rymer & Higham	*Preparing for the DRCoG*	1900603012
Sandler & Sandler	*MCQs in Cardiology for MRCP Pt I*	0792389999
Sandler & Sandler	*MCQs in Cardiology*	0792389387
Sandler & Sandler	*More MCQs in Cardiology for MRCP Pt I*	0792388402
Sikdar	*MCQs in Basic Sciences for MRCPsych Pt II*	190060356X

Obtainable from all good booksellers or, in case of difficulty, from Plymbridge Distributors Limited, Plymbridge House, Estover Road, PLYMOUTH, Devon PL6 7PZ
Tel.   01752–202300
Fax   01752–202333

Multiple-choice Questions on the Upper Digestive Tract

Edited by

Malcolm C. Bateson

Consultant Physician and Gastroenterologist
General Hospital, Bishop Auckland, County Durham, UK

and

Eighteen Teachers

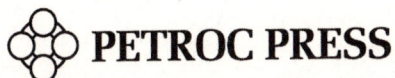 PETROC PRESS

Petroc Press, an imprint of LibraPharm Limited

Distributors
Plymbridge Distributors Limited, Plymbridge House, Estover Road, Plymouth PL6 7PZ, UK

Copyright
©1999 LibraPharm Limited

All rights reserved. No part of this publication may be reproduced, stored in a retrieval system, or transmitted in any form or by any means, electronic, mechanical, photocopying, recording or otherwise, without prior permission from the publishers.

While every attempt has been made to ensure that the information provided in this book is correct at the time of printing, the publisher, its distributors, sponsors and agents, make no representation, express or otherwise, with regard to the accuracy of the information contained herein and cannot accept any legal responsibility or liability for any errors or omissions that may have been made or for any loss or damage resulting from the use of the information.

Published in the United Kingdom by
LibraPharm Limited
3b Thames Court
High Street
Goring-on-Thames
READING
Berkshire
RG8 9AQ
UK

A catalogue record for this book is available from the British Library

ISBN 1 900603 37 3

Printed and bound in the United Kingdom by
MPG Books Limited, Victoria Square, Bodmin, Cornwall PL31 1EG

Contents

Preface   vi
Authors   vii

Questions   1
Answers   28

Preface

These multiple-choice questions have been composed to provide both examination practice and up-to-date medical information in the explanation of the answers.

They are suitable for clinical medical students, junior doctors, candidates for the MRCP, MRCS and MRCGP, and trainees in gastroenterology. They are designed to be of varying levels of difficulty, and this should lead to an enjoyable self-teaching experience. Do not be surprised if you cannot answer all of the questions – this is part of the learning process.

Read the instructions carefully. The questions have a stem and five possible responses. For most of them, any number of the five answers could be true or false, but for some only the best answer is requested, so that only one answer will be true.

Wrong answers lose marks in examinations, so get into the habit of only responding when you are completely sure or almost certain of the correct reply.

Bishop Auckland, 1999   M.C.B.

Authors

Malcolm C. Bateson (*Editor*)	Bishop Auckland General Hospital
Subrata Ghosh	Western General Hospital, Edinburgh
Ray Holden	Monklands Hospital, Airdrie
Pali Hungin	Centre for Health Studies, University of Durham
James Rose	Ayr General Hospital
Eric Boyd	Nevill Hall Hospital, Abergavenny
Dennis Burke	Cumberland Infirmary, Carlisle
A. Umar	Royal Victoria Infirmary, Newcastle upon Tyne
Kenneth Matthewson	Hexham General Hospital
James Cox	Wansbeck General Hospital, Northumberland
Sami Shimi	Ninewells Hospital, Dundee
David Nylander	Freeman Hospital, Newcastle upon Tyne
Oliver Eade	Borders General Hospital, Melrose
Derek Gillen	Gartnavel General Hospital, Glasgow
Keith George	Gartnavel General Hospital, Glasgow
Jan Freeman	Derby City General Hospital
B. A. S. Jayasekara	Ninewells Hospital, Dundee
Vicki Save	Ninewells Hospital, Dundee
Robert A. B. Wood	Ninewells Hospital, Dundee

Questions

Q1 Drugs with useful effects on gastrointestinal motibility include:

A. Cisapride
B. Domperidone
C. Erythromycin
D. Metoclopramide
E. Misoprostol

Q2 In the management of dyspepsia in adults:

A. Gastroscopy should be used in patients over 45 years
B. Gastroscopy should be used in patients under 45 years with weight loss, anaemia or dysphagia
C. Pre-treatment with H_2-receptor antagonists will not affect *Helicobacter pylori* testing
D. Pre-treatment with proton pump inhibitors (PPI) will not affect *H. pylori* testing
E. Whole blood near patient testing for *H. pylori* will reliably guide management

Q3 Duodenal biopsy will sometimes demonstrate an infective origin for symptoms. Which one of the following organisms is most likely to be found?

A. Amoebae
B. Candida
C. Giardia
D. Helicobacter
E. Leishmaniasis

Q4 Which one of the following drugs has the best action against *Helicobacter pylori*?

A. Ciprofloxacin
B. Thiabendazole
C. Nalidixic acid
D. Tinidazole
E. Spiramycin

Q5 In non-cardiac chest pain, which of these investigations are likely to be useful?

A. CT scan of chest
B. Gastroscopy
C. Barium swallow or meal
D. 24-hour oesophageal pH
E. Oesophageal manometry

Q6 Which is the best one of these management plans for a patient with spontaneous duodenal ulcer to achieve reliable rapid primary healing and long-term cure?

A. Cimetidine 800 mg daily for 4 weeks
B. Omeprazole, amoxycillin and metronidazole for 1 week
C. Bismuth chelate 240 mg twice daily for 4 weeks
D. Lansoprazole 30 mg daily for 1 month; clarithromycin and metronidazole for 1 week
E. Pantoprazole 40 mg daily for 4 weeks

Q7 Which of the following does the stomach secrete into its lumen?

A. Pepsin
B. Gastrin
C. Acid
D. Vitamin B_{12}
E. Mucus

Q8 The following drugs, which were approved for general use in the UK in the 1990s, are inhibitors of the gastric proton pump:

A. Astemizole
B. Pantoprazole
C Carvedilol
D. Lansoprazole
E. Omeprazole

Q9 What is the frequency of *H. pylori* infection in British children?

A. 1%
B. 10%
C. 30%
D. 50%
E. 100%

Q10 What is the prevalence of active *H. pylori* infection in the British adult population?

A. 5%
B. 15%
C. 25%
D. 45%
E. 75%

Q11 Vegans:

A. Eat no meat
B. Eat no meat or fish
C. Eat no meat, fish or dairy products
D. Are prone to anaemia
E. May become B_{12} deficient

Q12 Enteroscopy is an important investigation:

A. In the routine investigation of coeliac disease
B. For gastrinoma
C. In obscure anaemia with iron deficiency
D. For giardiasis
E. In tropical sprue

Q13 Deficiency of which one of the B vitamins is most likely to cause clinical problems in alcoholism?

A. B_{17}
B. B_6
C. B_1
D. B_{52}
E. B_{12}

Q14 Alcohol excess increases the risk of cancer of:

A. Mouth
B. Oesophagus
C. Stomach
D. Duodenum
E. Lung

Q15 True food allergy is:

A. Uncommon
B. Usually identified correctly by the patients themselves
C. Associated with asthma, eczema and hay fever
D. Investigated by a diet containing only lamb, rice, pears and water for 2 weeks
E. Effectively treated with oral dexamethasone

Q16 A high roughage diet is indicated as specific treatment for:

A. Oesophageal dysmotility
B. Peptic ulcer
C. Diverticular disease
D. Coeliac disease
E. Irritable bowel syndrome

Q17 Adenocarcinoma of the cardia of the stomach:

A. Has been steadily decreasing in incidence
B. Is caused by *H. pylori*
C. Has a worse prognosis than gastric cancer of the body and antrum
D. May arise from fundic gland polyps
E. Is unusual in Caucasians

Q18 Barrett's oesophagus:

A. Is a congenital lesion
B. Associated with high-grade dysplasia may harbour foci of invasive carcinoma
C. May be associated with *p53* protein over-expression at a late stage of carcinogenesis
D. May be ablated by photodynamic therapy via an endoscope
E. Associated with hiatus hernia is best treated by Nissen fundoplication

Q19 A 56-year-old woman presented with fluctuating dysphagia, mainly for solids, over a period of one and a half years. She described retrosternal discomfort on eating and a weight loss of half a stone. Over the last 6 months she has also had nocturnal coughing spells.

A. Oesophageal manometry should be the initial diagnostic step
B. The differential diagnosis would include pharyngeal paralysis
C. A CT scan of the thorax and abdomen would be diagnostic
D. Resting lower oesophageal sphincter pressure will be the most useful diagnostic information
E. A peptic stricture is the likeliest diagnosis

Q20 Predisposing factors for Candida oesophagitis include:

A. Methotrexate therapy
B. Progressive systemic sclerosis
C. Corticosteroid use
D. Azathioprine therapy
E. Diabetes mellitus

Q21 Markedly thickened gastric folds may be associated with:

A. Zollinger-Ellison syndrome
B. Cronkhite-Canada syndrome
C. Cytomegalovirus infection
D. Pernicious anaemia
E. Gastric lymphoma

Q22 Aggressive parenteral refeeding in cachectic patients may lead to:

A. Hypophosphataemia
B. Hypoglycaemia
C. Ventricular tachyarrhythmias
D. Wernicke's encephalopathy
E. Fluid depletion

Q23 Complications associated with central vein parenteral nutrition include:

A. Cholestatic liver disease
B. Cholestasis
C. Osteopenia
D. Microvascular pulmonary emboli
E. Aluminium depletion

Q24 Gastric stasis without a mechanical obstruction may be a feature of:

A. Insulin-dependent diabetes mellitus but not NIDDM
B. Systemic sclerosis
C. Depression
D. Amyloidosis
E. Small cell carcinoma of the lung

Q25 Gastric carcinoid tumours:

A. Commonly occur in Zollinger-Ellison syndrome not associated with MEN-1 syndrome
B. May be associated with prolonged treatment with proton pump inhibitors
C. Have a good prognosis and surgical resection is unnecessary
D. May be missed by routine endoscopic biopsies
E. Do not cause carcinoid syndrome

Q26 Zenker's diverticula:

A. Are congenital
B. Are best diagnosed by direct visualisation at endoscopy
C. Are an anaesthetic hazard
D. May be treated at endoscopy
E. May cause halitosis

Q27 A 54-year-old woman with a previous history of peptic ulcer disease, treated by Bilroth II gastrectomy 21 years ago, presented with sweating, nausea, flushing and palpitations about 20 minutes after eating. She had lost about half a stone in weight.

A. She should undergo an endoscopy
B. Dietary advice may be useful to alleviate her symptoms
C. Plasma glucose should be monitored for at least 4 hours after eating
D. Octreotide therapy may be useful
E. Surgical referral for a roux-en-Y gastrojejunostomy should be considered

Q28 Reflux of gastric acid into the lower oesophagus:

A. Causes tertiary peristalsis
B. Induces reflux salivation
C. Is associated with bronchodilatation
D. Decreases cricopharyngeal tone
E. Is normal in the upright position

Q29 Recurrent oral aphthous ulceration (RAU) is associated with:

A. Iron deficiency
B. Coeliac disease
C. Idiopathic colitis
D. Behçet's disease
E. Crohn's disease

Q30 In Barrett's oesophagus:

A. There is an increased incidence of squamous carcinoma
B. Neoplasia can only occur after the development of intestinal metaplasia
C. The development of an ulcer is associated with an increased risk of neoplasia
D. Prophylactic oesophagectomy may be indicated if biopsies reveal severe dysplasia
E. Surgical anti-reflux procedures lead to a reduction in the affected segment

Q31 In patients with diffuse vascular anomaly of the gastric antrum (watermelon stomach)

A. A previous diagnosis of antral gastritis has often been made
B. Massive haematemesis is a common presentation
C. Blood transfusion may be required
D. Endoscopic sclerotherapy may be of value
E. Hormone replacement should be avoided

Q32 The endoscopic appearances of the duodenum in coeliac disease includes:

A. A mucosal mosaic pattern
B. Aphthoid erosions
C. Scalloped fold margins
D. Mucosal clefts or grooves
E. Reduced number and height of folds

Q33 The body mass index (BMI)

A. Is height (cm) / weight (kg)
B. Is height (m) / weight (kg)
C. Is weight (kg) / height (m^2)
D. Indicates adequate nutrition in a patient when it is 15
E. Is of little value in patients over 80 years

Q34 In duodenal ulceration:

A. The rate of healing is related to the duration of acid suppression
B. The rate of healing is related to the degree of acid suppression
C. Healing cannot be achieved in *Helicobacter* eradication only
D. Endoscopic confirmation of healing is advised in most cases
E. Recurrent dyspepsia after successful *Helicobacter* eradication is most commonly caused by reinfection

Q35 Gastro-oesophageal reflux disease is linked with:

A. Increased low oesophageal pressure
B. Delayed gastric emptying
C. Reflux of gastric fluid
D. Altered oesophageal motility
E. Chronic cough

Q36 Symptoms of gastro-oesophageal reflux disease may be exacerbated by:

A. Mebeverine
B. Metoclopramide
C. Calcium channel blockers
D. Cisapride
E. Spicy foods

Q37 Barrett's oesophagus:

A. Is an inevitable progression from chronic reflux disease
B. Frequency and severity of symptoms are indications of disease
C. Long-standing heartburn is usually present
D. Can lead to adenocarcinoma
E. The prevalence reduces with age

Q38 In dyspepsia:

A. The community prevalence is 10%
B. 75% of sufferers will consult their GP
C. Severity of symptoms is the chief reason for consultation
D. Accounts for 1% of the GP workload
E. Non-consulters have a shorter history

Q39 Serum urea levels are:

A. Low in liver disease
B. High in dehydration
C. Low in starvation
D. High in renal failure
E. Low in gout

Q40 Important causes of benign oesophageal stricture are:

A. Aspirin
B. Hiatus hernia
C. Alendronate
D. Bleach self-poisoning
E. Non-steroidal anti-inflammatory drugs

Q41 The following drugs heal peptic ulcers:

A. Cimetidine
B. Ranitidine
C. Famotidine
D. Rabeprazole
E. Nizatidine

Q42 Nitroimidazole resistance in *H. pylori*:

A. Is transferable between organisms of different strains
B. Is equally common in male and female patients
C. Results in failure of eradication therapy in over 50% of patients treated with a triple regimen containing a nitroimidazole
D. Has a prevalence of 45% in UK populations
E. Should be routinely tested for in patients being considered for eradication therapy

Q43 Gastric metaplasia of the duodenal bulb:

A. Is colonised by *H. pylori* in more than 90% of patients with duodenal ulcer
B. Regresses in response to prolonged inhibition of gastric acid
C. Contains parietal and chief cells
D. Stains with the periodic acid Schiff's reagent
E. Is always pathological

Q44 When testing for the presence of *H. pylori*:

A. Tests to confirm eradication should be delayed for 28 days after completion of therapy
B. Serological tests are suitable for confirmation of eradication
C. The urea breath test is the most sensitive and specific non-invasive test
D. Both fundic and antral biopsies should be obtained at endoscopy in patients who are currently taking gastric anti-secretory drugs
E. The Warthin-Starry stain is specific for *H. pylori*

Q45 The development of anti-microbial resistance by *H. pylori* is a problem during treatment with:

A. Amoxycillin
B. Tetracycline
C. Metronidazole
D. Clarithromycin
E. Bismuth subcitrate

Q46 Recognised interactions of drugs used in the eradication therapy of *H. pylori* include:

A. Potentiation of warfarin by omeprazole and lansoprazole
B. Disulfiram reaction to alcohol with tinidazole
C. Cisapride-induced arrhythmias with clarithromycin
D. Increased absorption of bismuth when administered with ranitidine
E. Reduced effectiveness of tetracycline-containing regimens if antacids are taken simultaneously.

Q47 The Zollinger-Ellison syndrome:

A. May cause malabsorption of vitamin B_{12}
B. is usually a manifestation of the multiple endocrine adenomatosis (MEA) type 1 syndrome
C. Should initially be treated with proton pump inhibitor
D. Usually presents with ulceration involving the second and third parts of the duodenum
E. Results from a benign gastrinoma in more than 50% of cases

Q48 The *cag A* gene, when expressed by *H. pylori*:

A. Codes for a protein which stimulates parietal cell secretion
B. Does not result in a detectable humoral antibody response
C. Causes more rapid progression of chronic atrophic gastritis
D. Is associated with an increased risk of developing duodenal ulcer
E. Confers resistance to nitroimidazole antibacterials

Q49 The following are accepted stains for the demonstration of *H. pylori* in endoscopic gastric biopsies:

A. Alcian Blue
B. Giemsa
C. Congo Red
D. Warthin-Starry
E. Gram

Q50 Vomiting in infancy may be due to:

A. Gastro-oesophageal reflux
B. Hypertrophic pyloric stenosis
C. Cow's milk protein intolerance
D. Coeliac disease (gluten-sensitive enteropathy)
E. Hirschsprung's disease

Q51 *H. pylori*:

A. Is a Gram-positive obligate aerobe
B. Is not motile
C. Can be detected because of its ability to liberate ammonium ions from urea
D. Eradication improves the symptoms of gastro-oesophageal reflux
E. Sero-positivity is associated with alcohol abuse

Q52 A Pólya gastrectomy:

A. Avoids the complication of bacterial overgrowth
B. May be associated with bone disease
C. Can lead to the 'dumping syndrome'
D. Prevents gastro-oesophageal reflux
E. Does not cause iron deficiency anaemia

Q53   In the Zollinger-Ellison (ZE) syndrome:

A. Steatorrhoea may occur
B. Diarrhoea may be a feature
C. Hypogastrinaemia is due to atrophy of G-cells
D. Only duodenal ulceration occurs
E. Can be controlled by the use of proton pump inhibitors

Q54   In a 55-year-old patient with new onset positional and food-related dyspeptic symptoms:

A. A hiatal hernia is a prerequisite to confirm the diagnosis of gastro-oesophageal reflux disease (GORD)
B. If *H. pylori* sero-positive, indicates a peptic ulcer
C. Gastroscopy is advised
D. A normal endoscopy excludes acid-related dyspepsia
E. A pH level > 6 measured 5 cm above the gastro-oesophageal junction indicates gastro-oesophageal reflux

Q55   Achalasia of the cardia:

A. The majority of cases present in childhood
B. There is incomplete relaxation of the lower oesophageal sphincter (LOS) on swallowing
C. Patients may present with chronic cough
D. Occurs in scleroderma
E. Can be treated by pneumatic dilatation

Q56   Odynophagia may be caused by:

A. Herpetic oesophagitis
B. Oesophageal candidiasis
C. Gastro-oesophageal reflux
D. Cholelithiasis
E. Tetracycline

Q57   Gastric acid:

A. Is produced by the oxyntic cells in the stomach
B. Is reduced by sucralfate
C. Is utilised by *H. pylori* to produce ammonia
D. Secretion is stimulated by acetylcholine
E. Secretion is inhibited by omeprazole

Q58 Gastrointestinal haemorrhage:

A. Mortality is independent of age
B. The finding of a visible vessel in an ulcer base indicates a rebleeding rate of 25%
C. H_2-receptor antagonists reduce the risk of rebleeding from PU
D. May occur in patients with ectopic gastric mucosa
E. May arise from the watermelon stomach

Q59 The following drugs affect portal pressure:

A. Octreotide
B. Propranolol
C. Simvastatin
D. Vasopressin
E. Sucralfate

Q60 The following may be used to assess Barrett's oesophagus for malignancy:

A. Length
B. pH
C. Dysplasia
D. Mucin staining
E. Molecular staining

Q61 Symptoms of gastro-oesophageal reflux in children may typically include:

A. Failure to thrive
B. Irritability
C. Low thyroid stimulating hormone (TSH) levels
D. Epigastric pain
E. Stridor

Q62 Saliva:

A. About 750 ml is produced daily
B. The largest volume is produced by the parotid gland
C. Has a specific gravity similar to that of urine
D. Contains amino acids
E. Plays a greater role in speech than in swallowing

Q63 **Hypergastrinaemia may occur in:**

A. Chronic renal failure
B. Proton pump inhibitor (PPI) therapy
C. Shock
D. *H. pylori* infection
E. Carcinoid tumours

Q64 **In the stomach:**

A. Enterochromaffin-like (ECL) cells in the antrum synthesise histamine by the decarboxylation of histidine
B. ECL cells are present throughout the stomach
C. *H. pylori* infection can either increase or decrease acid output
D. Removal of saliva by suction increases acid clearance time
E. Trichobezoars occur almost exclusively in males

Q65 **Alteration in taste sensation may result from:**

A. Bell's palsy
B. Head injury
C. Turner's syndrome (sex chromosomes XO)
D. Thermal burn
E. Hepatic cirrhosis

Q66 **Recognised causes of haematemesis from upper gastrointestinal bleeding include:**

A. Para-oesophageal hiatus hernia
B. Dieulafoy's lesions
C. 'Water melon' stomach
D. Haemobilia
E. Sandblom's triad

Q67 **Gastric carcinoma may arise from:**

A. Chronic gastritis
B. Gastric polyps
C. Chronic peptic ulcer
D. Tylosis
E. Achalasia

Q68 The following will cause an increase in lower oesophageal sphincter activity:

A. Bombesin
B. Chocolate
C. Alcohol
D. Protein meal
E. Enkephalins

Q69 Oesophageal cancer:

A. Is becoming increasingly rare
B. Is usually curable by surgery
C. Is most commonly of the squamous cell type
D. May occur as a complication of chronic gastro-oesophageal reflux disease
E. Is usually treated by the insertion of a PEG (percutaneous endoscopic gastrostomy)

Q70 An 84-year-old woman with two previous myocardial infarctions presents with dysphagia for solids, and gives a long-standing history of heartburn. At endoscopy she is found to have Barrett's oesophagus and an oesophageal stricture.

A. The stricture is almost certainly benign
B. Oesophageal dilatation would be too high a risk procedure to perform
C. H_2-receptor antagonists would be an effective treatment
D. An oesophageal endoprosthesis (tube or stent) should be inserted immediately
E. 24-hour intra-oesophageal pH monitoring is indicated

Q71 The mortality rate in acute upper GI haemorrhage:

A. Is 11% in patients admitted to hospital with bleeding
B. Is over 50% if it arises in an in-patient
C. Is less than 0.5% in under 60-year-olds with no co-morbidity
D. Has fallen progressively in recent years with the introduction of more advanced intensive therapy
E. Is independent of the underlying cause

Q72 PEG insertion may be indicated in:

A. Motor neurone disease
B. Huntingdon's chorea
C. Cancer of the tongue
D. Cystic fibrosis
E. Chronic renal failure

Q73 PEG insertion is contra-indicated if:

A. The patient has a hiatus hernia
B. The patient has disseminated intra-abdominal malignancy
C. The prothrombin time is prolonged by 4 seconds or greater
D. The patient has intestinal obstruction
E. The patient has ascites

Q74 Achalasia of the cardia:

A. Is a disease of young people
B. Has a familial incidence
C. Is caused by loss of smooth muscle
D. Commonly presents as chest pain
E. Is best diagnosed at gastroscopy

Q75 Elevation of plasma gastrin is found in:

A. Zollinger-Ellison syndrome
B. Pernicious anaemia
C. Renal failure
D. Treatment with cimetidine
E. Hypocalcaemia

Q76 The following may increase the potential for carcinoma complicating Barrett's oesophagus:

A. Long length of gastric metaplasia
B. Presence of hiatus hernia
C. Use of anti-reflux surgery
D. Intestinal metaplasia
E. *H. pylori* infection

Q77 Drugs with useful effects on gastrointestinal motility include:

A. Cisapride
B. Domperidone
C. Erythromycin
D. Metoclopramide
E. Misoprostol

Q78 Which of the following statements are correct in dermatitis herpetiformis?

A. Rash is common on the buttocks
B. Rash is common on the face
C. Rash is itchy
D. Blisters are usually present
E. Pre-menstrual exacerbation may occur

Q79 Recognised features of coeliac disease include:

A. Vasculitis
B. Vitamin D deficiency
C. Haemarthrosis
D. Splenomegaly
E. Bacterial overgrowth

Q80 The following is true in Boerhaave's syndrome:

A. Antibiotics should always be given
B. Thoracotomy is best delayed until the patient has received an oesophageal washout
C. The sex instance is equal between men and women
D. Immediate endoscopy is mandatory
E. The pain usually radiates to the left hypochondrium or shoulder

Q81 The following statements are true of heartburn in pregnancy:

A. One of the causes is a decreased lower oesophageal sphincter
B. Gastric emptying is actually increased
C. Gastroscopy is crucial
D. It occurs in late pregnancy
E. It is relieved by delivery

Q82 In carcinoma of the oesophagus:

A. Tylosis is usual
B. Sub-mucosal spread is usual
C. Adenocarcinomas are now the most common cell type
D. Tracheo-oesophageal fistula is best treated by surgery
E. It is more common in caustic injury

Q83 Micro-angiopathic haemolytic anaemia is a recognised complication of:

A. Achalasia
B. Carcinoma of the stomach
C. Coeliac disease
D. Boerhaave's syndrome
E. Peutz-Jeghers' syndrome

Q84 The following features individually suggest achalasia as the cause of dysphagia:

A. Aperistalsis in the oesophagus on manometry
B. Dysphagia for solids and liquids
C. Bird's beak deformity on barium meal
D. Normal upper GI endoscopy
E. A narrow stricture in the lower oesophagus

Q85 The following factors are implicated in gastro-oesophageal reflux:

A. Caffeine intake
B. *H. pylori* eradication
C. Previous partial gastrectomy and Billroth I reconstruction
D. Glyceryl trinitrate (GTN) therapy
E. Stenting a benign lower oesophageal stricture

Q86 Resectability of cancer of the intra-thoracic oesophagus depends on:

A. The presence or absence of cervical lymph nodes
B. The length of the cancer
C. The presence or absence of diaphragmatic metastasis
D. The presence or absence of bronchiectasis
E. Previous radiotherapy to the chest

Q87 In Boerhaave's syndrome:

A. Oesophageal tear is caused by repeated coughing
B. Surgical management depends on the period from onset to presentation
C. Mediastinitis is caused by anaerobic organisms
D. The diagnosis is confirmed by barium swallow
E. The initial management involves nasogastric intubation

Q88 The following benign oesophageal conditions can cause non-cardiac chest pain:

A. Diffuse oesophageal spasm
B. High-amplitude peristaltic contractions
C. Achalasia
D. Gastro-oesophageal reflux without oesophagitis
E. Oesophagitis

Q89 In a 24-hour ambulatory pH recording from the oesophagus:

A. The pH probe is positioned at the oesophago-gastric junction
B. A reflux event is defined as a drop in pH below 4
C. The duration of reflux events defines oesophageal clearance
D. Can be used to determine duodeno-gastric reflux
E. The complete absence of reflux episodes indicate the presence of a peptic stricture

Q90 Barrett's metaplasia in the oesophagus:

A. Develops in a third of patients with chronic gastro-oesophageal reflux disease
B. Disappears after medical treatment using proton pump inhibitors
C. Disappears after surgical treatment by fundoplication
D. Can progress to dysplasia only if the metaplasia is of the intestinal type
E. In short segments, carries a lower malignant potential

Q91 The indications for radiotherapy in patients with oesophageal cancer include:

A. Pre-operatively without chemotherapy
B. Post-operatively after curative (R0) resection
C. Post-operatively after palliative resection
D. For patients with tracheo-bronchial fistula
E. For patients with bone metastases

Q92 The following drugs used singly are of established benefit in the healing of oesophagitis:

A. Cisapride
B. Omeprazole
C. Sucralfate
D. Metoclopramide
E. Ranitidine

Q93 Oesophageal diverticula:

A. Are commonly congenital
B. Give rise to dysphagia
C. Are commonly pulsion diverticula
D. Are usually associated with a motility disorder of the oesophagus
E. Only require excision if they cause significant mechanical disturbance

Q94 In coeliac disease:

A. There are reduced numbers of intra-epithelial lymphocytes in duodenal mucosal biopsy
B. The anti-endomysial antibody is likely to be positive in younger patients
C. There is an increased risk of squamous cell oesophageal carcinoma
D. First-degree relatives do not have an increased risk of having the condition
E. The prevalence is increased among insulin-dependent diabetes

Q95 Duodenal ulcer (DU)

A. Is associated with normal acid secretion
B. Is rarely related to Crohn's disease
C. Is more prevalent than gastric ulcers
D. Is usually found in the first part of the duodenum
E. Is a rare cause of upper GI haemorrhage

Q96 The following are true of proton pump inhibitors (PPIs)

A. Are competitive inhibitors of the proton pump
B. Are more effective in *H. pylori*-infected subjects
C. Increase the accuracy of *H. pylori* diagnostic tests
D. Are the treatment of choice for gastric ulcers
E. Undergo metabolism by cytochrome P450 pathways

Q97   Gastric ulcers:

A. Are mostly NSAID related
B. Are usually associated with low acid secretion
C. Are uncommonly malignant
D. Are the most common form of peptic ulcer
E. Are the commonest cause of upper GI haemorrhage

Q98   The gastric enterochromaffin-like (ECL) cell:

A. Inhibits parietal cell function
B. Has somatostatin as its main vesicle content
C. Is sensitive to gastrin's trophic effects
D. Is stimulated through H_2-receptors
E. Is the cell-type from which gastric carcinoma arises

Q99   There is a higher incidence of distal gastric carcinoma with:

A. High dietary salt
B. Post-gastrectomy
C. Coeliac disease
D. Pernicious anaemia
E. Duodenal ulcer disease

Q100 The following are true of distal gastric carcinoma:

A. *H. pylori* infection is an uncommon association
B. Hyposecretion of acid is common
C. Incidences are higher in South America
D. Incidences relative to proximal carcinoma are decreasing
E. Atrophic gastritis is frequently seen

Q101 The following are causes of *H. pylori*-negative duodenal ulcers:

A. Crohn's disease
B. Schistosomiasis
C. Coeliac disease
D. ACE inhibitors
E. Hyperparathyroidism

Q102 The following are reliable indicators of portal hypertension:

A. Gastric varices
B. Hereditary haemorrhagic telangiectasia
C. Dieulafoy's anomaly
D. 'Watermelon' stomach
E. Portal hypertensive gastropathy

Q103 Iron absorption in the upper GI tract:

A. Is less important than in the distal ileum
B. Is enhanced by acid suppression
C. Is enhanced by vitamin C
D. Is enhanced by tea
E. Is balanced by iron excretion

Q104 The risk of bleeding from oesophageal varices is increased:

A. If the hepatic venous pressure gradient is less than 10 mmHg
B. If varices are large
C. In Child-Pugh class A compared with class C
D. If bacterial infection is present
E. If alcohol excess ceases

Q105 Drugs used in primary prophylaxis against bleeding from oesophageal varices include:

A. Propranolol
B. Glypressin
C. Isosorbide mononitrate
D. Captopril
E. Atenolol

Q106 Which of the following statements about iron absorption are true?

A. The duodenum is the site of maximal iron absorption
B. Partial gastrectomy causes iron deficiency
C. Pernicious anaemia is associated with iron deficiency
D. Haem iron is more readily absorbed than non-haem iron
E. Haem iron accounts for the majority of absorbed iron

Q107 The following are true of *H. pylori* eradication therapy:

A. Amoxycillin resistance is a common problem
B. Antibiotic resistance is the most common cause of treatment failure
C. Side-effects are common
D. One week of treatment is recommended
E. The treatment of choice in *H. pylori*-positive non-ulcer dyspepsia

Q108 In the detection of *H. pylori* infection by the urease test, concomitant administration of drugs may cause problems as:

A. Antibacterials decrease the number of bacteria
B. Proton-pump inhibitors do not have direct antibacterial effects.
C. Proton-pump inhibitors inhibit the urease enzymes on which the test is based
D. Suppression of acid by proton-pump inhibitors causes the migration of *H. pylori* to the proximal stomach
E. Neutral acid pH can cause colonisation by *Proteus* spp., which produce urease

Q109 Mallory–Weiss tear:

A. Usually occurs in the mid-oesophagus
B. Usually causes life-threatening haemorrhage
C. Results in stricture of the oesophagus
D. Is a transmural tear
E. Is always a self-limiting haemorrhage

Q110 Oesophageal carcinoma:

A. Adenocarcinoma is the most common form of oesophageal carcinoma world-wide
B. Most adenocarcinomas arise in association with Barrett's oesophagus
C. Repeated balloon dilatation is the best form of palliative treatment for dysphagia in patients not suitable for surgery
D. Squamous carcinoma may develop in achalasia of the cardia owing to long-standing stasis
E. Can always be differentiated from benign stricture on barium swallow

Q111 Oesophageal dysmotility syndromes:

A. May present with chest pain indistinguishable from myocardial ischaemia
B. Corkscrew oesophagus on barium swallow suggests hypertensive peristalsis
C. Nutcracker oesophagus responds to treatment with β-blockers
D. Deployment of an expandable metal stent is the treatment of choice for achalasia of the cardia
E. Botulinum toxin injections may be used in the treatment of achalasia of the cardia

Q112 Branch chain amino acids:

A. As an infusion are effective in the treatment of hepatic encephalopathy
B. Include phenylalanine and tyrosine
C. As an infusion improve nitrogen balance in chronic liver disease
D. Are found in high concentrations in muscle
E. Act as a co-transporter of iron across the gut

Q113 Proton pumps are found in:

A. Myocytes
B. Renal tubules
C. Parietal cells
D. Colonic epithelia
E. Pancreatic acinar cells

Q114 Following a Pólya gastrectomy:

A. There is an increased risk of pulmonary tuberculosis
B. Megaloblastic anaemia, owing to folate deficiency, frequently occurs
C. H. pylori is eradicated
D. There is a decreased risk of gastric cancer
E. Metabolic bone disease is common

Q115 Total parenteral nutrition (TPN)

A. May cause jaundice
B. May cause pancreatitis
C. Should be used in the treatment of short bowel syndrome
D. May cause diarrhoea
E. May be admitted through a peripheral vein

Q116 Re-feeding under-nourished patients:

A. Increases metabolic rate
B. Causes serum levels of electrolytes to rise
C. May lead to cardiac and respiratory failure
D. Wernicke's encephalopathy may occur
E. Frequently causes constipation

Q117 In achalasia:

A. 20% of cases occur before the age of 14 years
B. There is an increased risk of oesophageal cancer
C. May present with nocturnal coughing
D. Retrosternal pain is a more common symptom in the elderly
E. Is adequately treated with cispride

Q118 The following drugs can cause oesophagitis:

A. Sucralfate
B. Tetracycline
C. Alendronate
D. Amoxycillin
E. Potassium chloride

Q119 Gastrin-secreting tumours leading to Zollinger-Ellison syndrome can be found in:

A. Bronchi
B. Pancreas
C. Ovary
D. Duodenal wall
E. Parathyroid gland

Q120 Iatrogenic disease of the gastrointestinal tract. Which of the following are true?

A. Slow-release potassium chloride preparations may be associated with multiple oesophageal ulcers
B. Anti-cholinergic agents may cause significant gastro-oesophageal reflux disease
C. Gastric ulcers induced by non-steroidal anti-inflammatory drugs (NSAIDs) characteristically occur in the body of the stomach, but these can be avoided by the use of suppositories
D. Malabsorption may be a complication of mefenamic acid
E. NSAIDs may give rise to a 'diaphragm' disease leading to recurrent sub-acute obstruction

Q121 Oral pigmentation may be related to:

A. Drugs
B. Ulcerative colitis
C. Hormonal imbalance
D. Tumours
E. Laxative abuse

Q122 Which of the following are true?

A. Oral manifestations of disease are more frequent in ulcerative colitis than in Crohn's disease
B. Haemoglobinopathies may cause splaying of the upper teeth
C. Pancreatic disease may be associated with sub-mandibular salivary gland enlargement
D. Macroglossia may be due to myelomatosis
E. Sjögren's syndrome may complicate chronic active hepatitis

Q123 Squamous carcinoma of the oesophagus:

A. Is a disease of high socio-economic status
B. Has a high incidence in China and Iran
C. May be associated with alcohol ingestion and smoking
D. Corrosive oesophageal strictures carry an increased risk of development of oesophageal carcinoma
E. Oesophageal reflux is classically associated with an increased risk of squamous carcinoma of the oesophagus

Q124 Which of the following statements are true of gastric secretion?

A. When gastric acid secretion is elevated after a meal, sufficient H^+ may be secreted to raise the pH of the systemic blood and make the urine acid
B. Acid secretion is stimulated by acetylcholine and gastrin by increasing intracellular calcium ions
C. Prostaglandins of the E series inhibit gastric secretion
D. Energy required for pumping H^+ out of the Paneth cells is by cyclic AMP
E. The gastric glands secrete about 1–1.5 litres of gastric juice per day

Q125 Which of the following statements are true of intrinsic factor (IF)?

A. It is glycoprotein with a molecular weight similar to albumin
B. Secretion is by parietal cells in the body of the stomach
C. Inadequate diet of cyanocobalamin is the usual cause of megaloblastic anaemia
D. Intrinsic factor cyanocobalamin complex binds to receptors in the jejunum
E. Trypsin is required for the absorptive process to be efficient

Q126 Which of the following statements are true of salivary glands and saliva?

A. The most important gland for the volume of secretion is the sub-mandibular gland
B. Vasoactive intestinal peptide (VIP) is a co-transmitter for the sympathetic nerves of salivary secretion
C. Saliva is normally hypotonic in contrast to serum
D. Parotid secretion is primarily a viscous secretion
E. The salivary secretion amounts to about 700 ml/24 h

Q127 Which of the following statements are true of swallowing?

A. The tractus solitarius and nucleus ambiguus are in the mid-brain
B. Afferent impulses are generated from receptors and passed via the trigeminal glossopharyngeal and vagus nerves
C. The glottic closure is caused by inhibition of respiration
D. The cricopharyngeus muscle relaxes reflexly upon swallowing
E. Food passes down the oesophagus at 10 cm/s

Answers

A1
A. True
B. True
C. True
D. True
E. False

Cisapride, metoclopramide and domperidone are all prokinetic agents which can be helpful in nausea, gastrointestinal reflux and some cases of irritable bowel.

A2
A. True
B. True
C. True
D. False
E. False

The PPI drugs have a specific action to suppress *Helicobacter pylori*, and may give rise to false-negative tests for this organism.

Whole blood testing is not accurate enough to be incorporated in management plans – urea breath test and ELISA serology are better tests.

A3
A. False
B. False
C. True
D. False
E. False

Giardia is the only organism which can commonly be demonstrated in the duodenum. It may occur in the epidermis in travellers, or be found where there is immune paresis, as in IgA deficiency.

A4
A. False
B. False
C. False
D. True
E. False

Regimens against *H. pylori* need at least two antibiotics to achieve satisfactory results. Antibiotic treatment for one week is optimal. Metronidazole and tinidazole are equally effective. Other first-choice antibiotics include clarithromycin, amoxycillin and tetracycline. Bismuth has anti-*H. pylori* activity, too. Bismuth chelate combined with PPI and two antibiotics, and ranitidine bismuth citrate combined with two antibiotics, are alternative useful regimens.

A5
A. False
B. True
C. True
D. True
E. True

Evaluation of non-cardiac chest pain is often unrewarding. Oesophagitis may be seen at endoscopy, and reflux without macroscopic change can be shown on pH monitoring. Simply testing people with omeprazole 40 mg bd. for a week will sometimes prove reflux, where symptoms are completely abolished.

Motility disorders may show on barium radiology – achalasia or corkscrew oesophagitis, but manometry is needed for more subtle changes.

A6
A. False
B. False
C. False
D. True
E. False

All of these treatments are quite effective and should achieve 80%+ primary healing. The PPIs are equivalent in efficacy, and a one-month treatment for primary healing is appropriate. H_2-receptor antagonists, such as cimetidine and ranitidine, are probably best given for 6–8 weeks.

Control, or preferably eradication, of *H. pylori* gives the best chance of long-term cure. Bismuth chelate will heal ulcers and reduce relapse. PPI plus antibiotic regimens are, however, the therapy of choice: clarithromycin and a nitro-imidazole or amoxycillin seem to be the most effective combinations. Use of PPI for a whole month probably improves the initial healing rate.

A7
A. True
B. False
C. True
D. False
E. True

The stomach secretes intrinsic factor which is necessary for the absorption of dietary B_{12}. Gastrin is a hormone secreted by the antrum into the bloodstream, from which it acts on the body of the stomach to stimulate acid secretion.

A8
A. False
B. True
C. False
D. True
E. False

The PPI drugs lansoprazole, pantoprazole and rabeprazole were introduced in 1994, 1996 and 1998, respectively. The PPI omeprazole has been in use since the 1980s, so experience is much more extensive.

Astemizole is an anti-histamine blocking H_2-receptor and free of sedative action. Carvedilol is a new β-blocker which may be especially useful in heart failure.

A9
A. False
B. True
C. False
D. False
E. False

About one in ten children have positive ELISA serology, and this is age dependent. If children have persistent dyspepsia and are *H. pylori* positive, then anti-Helicobacter therapy is appropriate.

A10
A. False
B. False
C. False
D. True
E. False

Population surveys by ELISA serology and endoscopy surveys of patients with normal upper GI tracts show that about half of adults carry *H. pylori*. This is age related, increasing up to 70 years. However, only 10% of the population is subject to peptic ulcer disease.

A11
A. False
B. False
C. True
D. True
E. True

Both vegetarians (who eat dairy products) and vegans (who do not) are prone to iron deficiency and may require supplementation.

Dietary vitamin B_{12} is derived from animal sources. There is a risk of B_{12} deficiency in vegans leading to anaemia and nerve damage, which can occur independently of each other.

A12
A. False
B. False
C. True
D. False
E. False

In iron-deficient anaemia where gastroscopy, duodenal biopsy and large bowel investigations are negative, enteroscopy may show angiodysplasia or small bowel ulcers. This is particularly useful in patients on non-steroidal anti-inflammatory drugs, where diaphragms also occur.

All the other conditions should be diagnosable by ordinary upper digestive endoscopy, duodenal biopsy and blood tests.

A13
A. False
B. False
C. True
D. False
E. False

Thiamine (B$_1$) deficiency may cause wet beriberi (heart failure), dry beriberi (peripheral neuropathy) and encephalopathies such as Korsakoff psychosis (amnesia and confabulation) and Wernicke's encephalopathy (confusion and ophthalmoplegia). However, complex deficiencies are common, including riboflavin, folic acid, pyridoxine and nicotinic acid. Unlike other B vitamins, B$_{12}$ is stored in large amounts, so shortage is unlikely.

A14
A. True
B. True
C. True
D. False
E. False

There is probably a direct toxic effect, more prominent for the proximal GI tract, but also seen for the stomach. Primary liver cancer is another important relationship.

A15
A. True
B. False
C. True
D. True
E. False

Patients often ascribe gastrointestinal symptoms to the foods they eat, but are usually wrong. There is an association between atopy and food allergy, which may be further investigated by skin prick tests for suspect food, and serum RAST testing. However, false-positives are a problem. Only exclusion of the food to which intolerance occurs is acceptable management where food allergy can be proven.

A16
A. False
B. False
C. True
D. False
E. False

High roughage regimens and bulking agents such as ispaghula husk and methyl cellulose are indicated for diverticular disease. Their usefulness in other diseases is not established and they are best avoided except in constipation. Some patients report a definite deterioration in symptoms on high-roughage regimens, and also these need modification to exclude gluten if they are used in patients with coeliac disease.

A17
A. False
B. False
C. True
D. False
E. False

The incidence of adenocarcinoma of the cardia has increased in the past several decades, unlike carcinoma of other parts of the stomach which are on the decline. *H. pylori* infection rates in cardia cancer are lower than for cancer elsewhere in the stomach. Adenocarcinoma of the cardia carries a worse prognosis than tumours elsewhere in the stomach, as hepatic and lymph node metastasis are common at diagnosis. There is a marked predominance of white men in cardia cancer. Fundic gland polyps may occur in association with familial adenomatous polyposis, but are not a risk factor for gastric carcinoma.

A18
A. False
B. True
C. False
D. True
E. False

Though there is some controversy in definition, Barrett's oesophagus is metaplastic columnar epithelium lining the distal oesophagus that predisposes to the development of adenocarcinoma. Specialised intestinal metaplasia is the histological feature most associated with the risk of development of adenocarcinoma. Perhaps the term 'Barrett's oesophagus' should be discarded and replaced by 'columnar-lined oesophagus with or without specialised intestinal metaplasia'. In patients found to have high-grade dysplasia in Barrett's oesophagus with no tumour mass on initial endoscopy, one-third will already harbour foci of invasive cancer. Over-expression of mutant *p53* protein is an early event in carcinogenesis in specialised intestinal metaplasia, unlike colon cancer where it is a late event. Photodynamic therapy via endoscopy may ablate specialised intestinal metaplasia and eradicate dysplasia and early cancers. There is no convincing evidence that a surgical anti-reflux procedure will reverse specialised intestinal metaplasia.

A19
A. False
B. False
C. False
D. False
E. False

Though manometry will give useful diagnostic information, an endoscopy is mandatory in the investigation of dysphagia and weight loss. Pharyngeal palsy causes dysphagia initially with liquids, and nasal regurgitation. A CT scan is useful to stage oesophageal carcinoma, but the diagnostic value in dysphagia is limited. The history is suggestive of achalasia where incomplete relaxation of the lower oesophageal sphincter on swallowing is diagnostic, not resting sphincter characteristics. A peptic stricture is often preceded by a history of heartburn and the dysphagia is gradually progressive not fluctuating, often with little weight loss.

A20
A. False
B. True
C. True
D. False
E. True

Corticosteroids contribute to fungal infection by suppressing both lymphocyte and granulocyte function. Topical corticosteroids for asthma may lead to oropharyngeal and oesophageal candidiasis. Azathioprine and methotrexate are seldom associated with oesophageal candidiasis. Diabetes mellitus, adrenal dysfunction, alcoholism, old age, broad-spectrum antibiotics, AIDS and haematological malignancies are common predisposing factors for Candida oesophagitis. Poor oesophageal peristalsis, such as in progressive systemic sclerosis, predisposes to fungal oesophagitis.

A21
A. True
B. True
C. True
D. False
E. True

Zollinger-Ellison syndrome is associated with thick folds in the fundus and body of the stomach. Cronkhite-Canada syndrome is associated with GI polyposis, alopecia, nail dystrophy, pigmentation, weight loss and diarrhoea. The histology of gastric folds is similar to Ménétrièr's disease, an exceptionally rare disease with giant gastric folds and protein loss. In childhood Ménétrièr's disease, cytomegalovirus gastropathy is the likely cause. Gastric mucosal lymphoid tissue lymphoma causes mucosal fold thickening. Pernicious anaemia is associated with severe atrophic gastritis.

A22
A. True
B. False
C. True
D. True
E. False

During starvation, phosphate requirements are decreased because of the predominant use of fat as a fuel. Refeeding stimulates insulin release and intracellular uptake of phosphate. Phosphate is required for protein synthesis and extracellular phosphate concentration may fall. Hypophosphataemia is associated with muscle weakness, paraesthesia, seizures, coma and cardiopulmonary decompensation. During starvation, the ability of insulin to stimulate glucose uptake is impaired and thus refeeding with large amounts of parenteral glucose may lead to hyperglycaemia and even hyperosmolar coma. Carbohydrate refeeding in patients with thiamine depletion may precipitate Wernicke's encephalopathy. Ventricular tachyarrhythmias may occur during the first week of refeeding. Chronic under-nutrition is associated with decreased cardiac mass, and parenteral nutrition may lead to fluid overload and congestive cardiac failure; fluid depletion is uncommon unless hyperosmolar coma owing to hyperglycaemia is allowed to occur.

A23
A. True
B. True
C. True
D. True
E. False

Hepatic abnormalities are the most common GI complications associated with parenteral nutrition. Excessive glucose calories are often implicated and lack of enteral nutrition may lead to gallbladder sludge and cholelithiasis. Hepatic histology may show steatosis, steatohepatitis and cholestasis. Osteopenia may be observed in patients receiving parenteral nutrition for more than three months – several mechanisms have been proposed including aluminium toxicity, vitamin D toxicity and negative calcium balance caused by amino acid-induced hypercalciuria. Microvascular pulmonary emboli may occur related to particulate material and in-line filters should always be used.

A24
A. False
B. True
C. True
D. True
E. True

Prevalence of gastric stasis is similar for IDDM and NIDDM. Infiltrative processes, such as systemic sclerosis and amyloidosis, may cause gastric stasis, the latter also via autonomic neuropathy. Gastric stasis may be the presenting feature of psychiatric illnesses such as depression and eating disorders, and treatment by antidepressants may contribute to gastric stasis. The recent onset of gastric stasis in middle-aged or elderly patients with a history of smoking should alert the physician to a para-neoplastic disorder associated with small-cell lung cancer. The chest radiograph may be negative and IgG antibody directed against myenteric neurons may be detectable.

A25
A. False
B. False
C. False
D. True
E. False

Patients with Zollinger-Ellison syndrome are only at increased risk of developing gastric carcinoid tumours if they have associated multiple-endocrine neoplasia-1 (MEN-1) syndrome. Proton-pump-inhibitor-induced hypergastrinaemia is not documented to have caused gastric carcinoid tumour, but may cause enterochromaffin-like (ECL) cellular hyperplasia. Long-standing pernicious anaemia or atrophic gastritis may be associated with gastric carcinoid tumours. Complete excision should be attempted whenever possible, either by surgical or endoscopic resection. Gastric carcinoids synthesise various neuroendocrine peptides and can cause a distinctive carcinoid syndrome, but only after hepatic metastasis. Because of their submucosal location, up to 50% of routine endoscopic biopsies may be negative.

A26
A. False
B. False
C. True
D. True
E. True

Zenker's diverticula are acquired and present typically in the seventh and eighth decades of life. They develop through a defect between the inferior pharyngeal constrictor and the cricopharyngeal sphincter. The diagnosis is best confirmed by a barium swallow. To avoid aspiration, Zenker's diverticula should be emptied prior to induction of anaesthesia. Surgical treatment is recommended for symptomatic diverticula, but in poor anaesthetic-risk patients endoscopic treatment by cricopharyngeal myotomy is being increasingly used. Symptoms include regurgitation, aspiration, hoarseness of voice, halitosis and a gurgling noise on eating.

A27
A. True
B. True
C. False
D. True
E. False

Early dumping syndrome occurs 15–30 minutes after eating owing to unregulated gastric emptying and rapid fluid shifts. Adenocarcinoma may occur in the gastric stump after partial gastrectomy and symptoms such as nausea or epigastric discomfort require endoscopic inspection. Hypoglycaemia is a feature of late dumping syndrome occurring 2–4 hours after eating. Dietary advice to reduce carbohydrate intake, sweets and fluid intake with meals may be sufficient treatment in many patients. If patients do not respond to dietary measures, octreotide injections are highly effective. It is, however, expensive and needs daily injections – newer long acting preparations (lanreotide) may be more practical. Surgical therapy should hardly ever be required after the availability of octreotide.

A28
A. False
B. True
C. False
D. False
E. True

The lower oesophageal sphincter reflexes to allow the passage of food but also spontaneously in the upright position permitting venting of excess gas (so-called transient lower oesophageal sphincter relaxation – TLOSR). When acid refluxes into the lower gullet a number of protective reflexes occur. The volume is removed by secondary peristalsis (tertiary contractions are spontaneous), the acid is neutralised by increased alkaline salivation, and cricopharyngeus and the bronchi constrict.

A29
A. True
B. True
C. True
D. True
E. True

RAU is associated with haematinic deficiency of whatever cause as well as inflammatory diseases which affect the bowel. In Crohn's disease the mouth can also be affected by a granulomatous process, considered by many to be oral Crohn's disease, but also occurring independently as oro-facial granulomatosis.

A30
A. False
B. True
C. True
D. True
E. False

Barrett's oesophagus is the transformation of the oesophageal squamous epithelium into glandular epithelium, which is initially gastric in type. Progressive changes can occur, involving the intestinal metaplasia type, followed by increasingly severe dysplasia before neoplasia develops. Ulceration of the abnormal mucosa is associated with an increased risk of cancer. Reduction in the length of the metaplastic segment with any conventional therapy has yet to be demonstrated convincingly. Small cancers often co-exist with severe dysplasia and can be treated by oesophagectomy.

A31
A. True
B. False
C. True
D. True
E. False

Diffuse antral vascular anomalies produce red engorged streaks, which may become confluent. This appearance is often initially mistaken for severe gastritis. Patients usually present with an iron deficiency anaemia or occasionally a coffee ground vomit. Endoscopic treatment with diathermy, laser and sclerotherapy reduce blood loss, as does HRT.

A32
A. True
B. False
C. True
D. True
E. True

Although ulceration occurs in coeliac disease, it does so in the form of the rare ulcerative jejunitis. The presence of erosions would suggest an inflammatory condition such as Crohn's disease.

A33
A. False
B. False
C. True
D. False
E. False

The BMI provides a rough and universally applicable index to adult nutritional status by correcting the weight for the height of the patient. As the BMI falls below 19, patients are considered to be increasingly malnourished.

A34
A. True
B. True
C. False
D. False
E. False

With acid suppressants, ulcer healing is achieved by a combination of degree and duration of acid suppression; less potent agents take longer, and vice versa. Eradication of Helicobacter alone is sufficient to allow ulcers to heal, but additional healing agents may be felt advisable in some circumstances, e.g. after a bleed. In uncomplicated ulcers confirmation of healing is not required in the asymptomatic patient. Re-infection and recrudescence rates after successful eradication treatment, as evidenced by a negative breath test one month after completion, are very low and recurrent dyspepsia is usually due to some other cause – usually reflux.

A35
A. False
B. True
C. True
D. True
E. True

This is a major cause of chronic cough.

A36
A. True
B. False
C. True
D. False
E. True

Mebeverine enhances reflux by lowering low oesophageal tone. Metoclopramide and cisapride aid gastric emptying and increase lower oesophageal pressure.

A37
A. False
B. False
C. True
D. True
E. False

Barrett's oesophagus affects 10–15% of patients with oesophagitis.

A38
A. False
B. False
C. False
D. False
E. False

The actual prevalence is greater than 25%. 25% of these will consult their GP. Perceptions and fears of consequences is the chief reason for seeking medical advice. Dyspepsia accounts for about 5% of workload. There is no difference between consulters and non-consulters.

A39
A. True
B. True
C. True
D. True
E. False

Urea is synthesised in the liver from nitrogen largely derived from dietary protein. It is excreted by the kidneys, and in renal failure both serum urea and creatinine are raised. In dehydration the urea rises disproportionately to creatinine. Gout may be associated with raised urate levels.

A40
A. False
B. True
C. True
D. True
E. False

Because hiatus hernia is a cause of significant reflux in some patients, it is associated with peptic strictures, though it may be difficult to demonstrate after they have occurred. Both alkalis such as bleach, and biphosphates such as alendronate, can cause direct toxic damage to the oesophagus. Neither aspirin nor NSAIDs are known to cause oesophageal inflammation and stricture; indeed, NSAIDs may be protective.

A41
A. True
B. True
C. True
D. True
E. True

Cimetidine, ranitidine, nizatidine and famotidine are equivalent H_2-receptor antagonists, though there is still some debate over ideal dosage and duration of treatment. Rabeprazole is a new proton-pump inhibitor, probably equivalent to lansoprazole, pantoprazole and omeprazole.

A42
A. True
B. False
C. False
D. True
E. False

Unfortunately resistance is readily transferable between strains, and between *H. pylori* and other organisms.

Female patients are much more likely to be colonised by nitroimidazole-resistant *H. pylori*, because of the more frequent use of nitroimidazoles as single drug therapy for genital infections.

Although eradication rates are lower in patients colonised with nitroimidazole-resistant *H. pylori*, the overall failure rate is much less than 50%.

Nitroimidazole resistance rates vary geographically and approach 100% in parts of Africa.

This is not necessary. Studies of nitroimidazole resistance may be indicated in patients who have previously had an unsuccessful course of eradication therapy; and periodically in the endoscopy population to document changes in local prevalence of resistance.

A43
A. False
B. True
C. False
D. True
E. False

H. pylori can only be detected in duodenal biopsies of about 60% of patients with duodenal ulcers. Duodenal colonisation by *H. pylori* may not, therefore, be a prerequisite for the development of duodenal ulcer.

Duodenal gastric metaplasia becomes more extensive in response to chronic gastric hypersecretion, and has been demonstrated to regress following vagotomy or prolonged treatment with gastric anti-secretory drugs.

The presence of these cells indicates gastric 'heterotopia' (a different entity from gastric metaplasia).

The gastric mucosal cells stain positively for mucins.

Some degree of gastric metaplasia (approximately 5%) is a normal finding in the first-part of the duodenum.

A44
A. True
B. False
C. True
D. True
E. False

If patients are tested before 28 days, false-negative tests may result from *suppression* of *H. pylori* rather than from *eradication*.

Serological tests are only reliable for the confirmation of previous colonisation with *H. pylori*. After successful eradication therapy, raised antibody titres may take many months to fall, and in some patients may remain significantly elevated indefinitely.

During treatment with anti-secretory drugs, *H. pylori* may migrate from the antral to the fundic mucosa. The likelihood of a false-negative result is reduced by taking both antral and fundic biopsies.

The Warthin-Starry stain is not specific for *H. pylori*: other spiral gastric bacteria also stain positively (e.g. *Helicobacter heilmanni*, previous known as *Gastrospirillium hominis*).

A45
A. False
B. False
C. True
D. True
E. False

Although strains for *H. pylori* can be produced under experimental conditions which demonstrate resistance to amoxycillin or tetracycline, this has not been a problem in therapy with combination regimens.

The development of resistance to nitroimidazoles and macrolides does occur in clinical practice.

H. pylori does not become resistant to bismuth (Bi) preparations, and co-prescription of Bi will reduce the chances of *H. pylori* developing resistance to nitroimidazoles or macrolides.

A46
A. True
B. True
C. True
D. True
E. True

Omeprazole and lansoprazole inhibit hepatic mixed-function oxidase and potentiate the effects of warfarin.

All nitroimidazoles may cause a disulfiram ('Antabuse')-like reaction with alcohol, although the risks are over-estimated: small amounts of alcohol seldom cause problems.

In the normally secreting stomach, Bi reacts with HCl to form the insoluble oxychloride, so that systemic absorption of Bi is low. When Bi salts are given together with gastric anti-secretory drugs, systemic absorption of Bi is significantly increased, so this combination of drugs (for example, ranitidine bismuth citrate 'Pylorid') should be avoided for repeated or long-term use.

Antacids bind with tetracyclines, reducing bioavailability and effectiveness.

A47
A. True
B. False
C. True
D. False
E. False

Normally pancreatic proteases split B_{12}–R factor complexes formed at the low pH in the stomach, freeing B_{12} to combine with intrinsic factor at the higher pH of the duodenum. The low intra-duodenal pH resulting from gastric hypersecretion of acid inactivates pancreatic proteases and lowers pH to a level at which free B_{12} will not combine with IF. This may result in B_{12} malabsorption.

Most gastrinomas (about 80%) occur as an isolated phenomenon and are not part of the MEA type 1 syndrome.

PPIs are the best way of getting symptoms rapidly under control. Note that a high proportion of DUs in the Zollinger-Ellison syndrome are *H. pylori* negative.

Severe distal ulceration is, in fact, rare. The most common presentation is as a bulbar DU which either fails to heal, or relapses rapidly after apparently effective treatment. All such cases should raise the possibility of Zollinger-Ellison syndrome.

Most (60–80%) of gatrinomas are malignant, although tumour growth may be slow and metastasis late.

A48
A. False
B. False
C. True
D. True
E. False

The *cag A* gene (cytotoxin-associated gene) is not present (or not expressed) in all strains of *H. pylori*. When present, it is associated with increased pathogenicity, reflected in a greater likelihood of the development of duodenal ulcers, more rapid progression of superficial gastritis to atrophy, and an increased risk of gastric cancer. *Cag A* inhibits acid secretion in cell cultures.

Antibodies to *cag A* can be detected in patient's serum.

Cag A is unrelated to the presence for nitroimidazole resistance.

A49
A. False
B. True
C. False
D. True
E. True

The modified Giemsa stain is easy to perform and widely used. The Warthin-Starry silver stain is very sensitive but technically demanding. *H. pylori* stains Gram positive but Gram staining is regarded as relatively insensitive. *H. pylori* can be detected in haematoxylin and eosin (H&E)-stained gastric biopsies, but again the sensitivity is lower than when using the Giemsa or Warthin-Starry methods.

Alcian Blue is a stain for mucin, used in the evaluation of gastric dysplasia and gastric metaplasia of the duodenal bulb.

Congo Red is a stain used for the detection of amyloid.

A50
A. True
B. True
C. True
D. True
E. True

Vomiting is a common symptom of illness in infancy. Although coeliac disease and cow's milk protein intolerance affect the small bowel, leading to malabsorption, they frequently have vomiting. Hirschsprung's disease leads to intestinal obstruction.

A51
A. False
B. False
C. True
D. False
E. False

H. pylori is a Gram-negative microaerophilic curved rod. It has flagella enabling its motility. The pH change associated with the liberation of ammonium ions by the action of urease produced by *H. pylori* is the basis of the biopsy urease test.

A52
A. False
B. True
C. True
D. False
E. False

Bone disease and iron deficiency can both occur in Pólya gastrectomy and the cause is probably multifactorial: decreased intake (of calcium, vitamin D and iron), rapid transit and decreased acid leading to malabsorption. Reflux can still occur, but this may be alkaline secondary to bile reflux. Bacterial overgrowth can occur because of a 'blind loop'.

A53
A. True
B. True
C. False
D. False
E. True

Diarrhoea and steatorrhoea can occur in the ZE syndrome which results in hypergastrinaemia from a gastrinoma. The symptoms can be controlled by PPI.

A54
A. False
B. False
C. True
D. False
E. False

In new dyspepsia over 45 years, gastroscopy is advised. 50% of 50-year-olds are *H. pylori* sero-positive and this does not equate with peptic ulcer. pH < 4 for more than 10.5% of the time is indicative of GORD and gastroscopy can be normal.

A55
A. False
B. True
C. True
D. False
E. True

Only 5% of patients with achalasia present before age 15. Cough and other respiratory complications may occur owing to overspill into the airways from the dilated oesophagus. In scleroderma the LOS decreases.

A56
A. True
B. True
C. True
D. False
E. True

Tetracycline can cause oesophageal ulceration, which like herpes, Candida and reflux oesophagitis, can all lead to pain on swallowing. Biliary colic can present as chest pain but not odynophagia.

A57
A. False
B. False
C. False
D. True
E. True

Parietal cells produce gastric acid. Gastrin, histamine and acetylcholine stimulate the acid pump. Sucralfate does not affect gastric acid secretion but has mucosal protective properties. *H. pylori* produces ammonia from urea.

A58
A. False
B. False
C. False
D. True
E. True

Mortality rate increases with age, particularly those over 60. The rebleeding rate from ulcers with a visible vessel is in excess of 50%. H_2-receptor antagonists do not affect rebleeding rate.

A59
A. True
B. True
C. False
D. True
E. False

Simvastatin is a lipid-lowering drug which inhibits HMG CoA reductase. Octreotide is a somatostatin analogue which reduces portal pressure. Sucralfate has no effect on portal pressure but has been used to treat sclerotherapy-induced ulceration.

A60
A. True
B. False
C. True
D. True
E. True

For practical purposes, a length greater than 7 cm and actual dysplasia are important predictors of malignant potential.

A61
A. False
B. True
C. False
D. False
E. False

Although failure to thrive and stridor may be associated with gastro-oesophageal reflux, they are not typical in children. Epigastric pain is only a feature in adults.

A62
A. True
B. False
C. False
D. True
E. False

Large volumes are produced by a variety of glands. This is an important lubricant, initiates starch digestion and neutralises gastric acid in the oesophagus.

A63
A. True
B. True
C. False
D. True
E. True

The mechanisms are different, e.g. PPI therapy suppresses gastric acid secretion, which in turn disinhibits gastrin release. This is analogous to the hypergastrinaemia of pernicious anaemia, which is always associated with achlorhydria so benign peptic ulceration cannot occur.

In contrast, the hypergastrinaemia of chronic renal failure and carcinoid syndrome may well predispose to ulcers.

A64
A. False
B. True
C. True
D. True
E. False

ECL cells are present only in the body of the stomach.
Trichobezoars are almost exclusive to females and are often associated with a psychiatric disorder.

A65
A. True
B. True
C. True
D. True
E. True

A66
A. True
B. True
C. True
D. True
E. False

Sandblom's triad consists of melaena (not haematemesis), biliary pain and jaundice. Dieulafoy lesions are angiodysplasias.

A67
A. True
B. True
C. True
D. False
E. False

Tylosis and achalasia are associated with oesophageal carcinoma.

A68
A. True
B. False
C. False
D. True
E. False

Chocolate, alcohol and enkephalins lower oesophageal sphincter activity.

A69
A. False
B. False
C. False
D. True
E. False

The incidence of oesophageal cancer is increasing at the rate of approximately 10% per annum, with the increase being due to the adenocarcinoma variety which is now more common than the squamous type. The majority of patients are not amenable to surgery because the tumour is too advanced at the time of presentation. Barrett's oesophagus, a complication of chronic gastro-oesophageal reflux, may be further complicated by the development of dysplasia and then invasive malignancy. Although PEGs are occasionally used in patients with oesophageal cancer, it is more usual to insert a prosthetic tube endoscopically or give endoscopic laser therapy.

A70
A. False
B. False
C. False
D. False
E. False

This patient has had chronic gastro-oesophageal reflux and has developed Barrett's change. The stricture could be either benign due to the reflux disease or malignant as a complication of the Barrett's change, and biopsies are essential. Oesophageal dilatation should be performed to relieve her symptoms. A proton-pump inhibitor should be used as these are the only agents demonstrated to reduce the restenosis rate in benign oesophageal stricture.

An endoprosthesis should not be inserted as the nature of the stricture is not yet known. 24-hour pH monitoring would add nothing to this patient's management as the diagnosis of gastro-oesophageal reflux is clear.

A71
A. True
B. False
C. True
D. False
E. False

If bleeding arises in a patient already hospitalised with another diagnosis, the mortality rate is 35%. The mortality rate depends on age and co-morbidity. A fit, under 60-year-old with no serious co-morbidity has a mortality risk of 0.1%. The overall mortality rate has not fallen, probably because of the increasing age of affected patients. The mortality rate is particularly high in patients bleeding from varices.

A72
A. True
B. True
C. True
D. True
E. True

Patients with bulbar palsy from motor neurone disease often require PEG insertion to maintain nutrition and reduce the risk of aspiration. Huntingdon's chorea patients may have a daily calorific requirement of 5000 kcal/day because of the choreiform movements. They also develop swallowing problems, and PEG nutrition may be useful. PEG nutrition may be used as either a temporary peri-operative or permanent measure to maintain nutrition in patients with oro-pharyngeal cancer.

Although cystic fibrosis patients can swallow normally, they malabsorb and overnight feeding using a PEG tube can improve their nutritional status, particularly prior to lung transplantation.

Patients with severe chronic diseases may become malnourished and PEG feeding may be helpful.

A73
A. False
B. True
C. True
D. True
E. True

A PEG may safely be inserted in hiatus hernia patients as long as most of the stomach is below the diaphragm providing the guiding endoscopy can trans-illuminate the anterior abdominal wall. Disseminated intra-abdominal malignancy, abnormal clotting, intestinal obstruction and ascites are all contra-indications. Abnormal clotting should be reversed. Ascites between the gastric and abdominal wall will prevent the introducing cannula reaching the stomach.

A74
A. False
B. False
C. False
D. True
E. False

Achalasia usually presents in the middle years of life and is caused by loss of the mesenteric plexus. About one-third to one-half of patients have chest pain. The condition is readily diagnosed by a variety of methods, but milder cases may require manometry.

A75
A. True
B. True
C. True
D. True
E. False

Gastrin hypersecretion is the hallmark of the ZE syndrome. It is seen in the achlorhydria of pernicious anaemia and the hypochlorhydria of H_2-receptor antagonist treatment as a secondary effect. Raised levels also occur in renal failure. Raised serum calcium stimulates acid secretion.

A76
A. True
B. False
C. False
D. True
E. False

Barrett's oesophagus segments of 7 cm or longer are more prone to malignancy, and also intestinal metaplasia may be a precursor.

A77
A. True
B. True
C. True
D. True
E. False

Cisapride, metoclopramide and domperidone are all prokinetic agents which can be helpful in nausea, gastrointestinal reflux, and in some cases of irritable bowel syndrome and functional dyspepsia. Metoclopramide should be avoided under in those under 20 years because of the prevalence of Parkinsonian side-effects. Erythromycin also influences motility and can be effective in diabetic gastroparesis; higher doses do, however, cause marked gastrointestinal side-effects. Misoprostol is a gastric mucosal protective agent and weak anti-acid, but effective doses are frequently limited by diarrhoea.

A78
A. True
B. True
C. True
D. False
E. True

The rash occurs in some two-thirds of patients on their buttocks, and the facet is a common site. The rash is itchy, and scratching tends to disrupt blisters.

A79
A. True
B. True
C. True
D. False
E. True

Fat-soluble vitamin deficiency, including vitamin K, occurs with steatorrhoea, and this may cause haemarthrosis. Usually the spleen is small and up to one-third may have bacterial overgrowth.

A80
A. True
B. False
C. False
D. False
E. True

Antibiotic treatment is mandatory but an oesophageal washout and early endoscopy would be extremely dangerous. It is five times more common in men.

A81
A. True
B. False
C. False
D. True
E. True

Gastric emptying is delayed because of the large uterus. Endoscopy is not usually necessary or wise. Although heartburn often occurs in early pregnancy, it also occurs in late pregnancy.

A82
A. False
B. True
C. False
D. False
E. True

Tylosis is a recognised association but is rare. Sub-mucosal spread is common. Squamous cell carcinoma is the commonest type, with adenocarcinoma increasing. Tracheo-oesophageal fistula implies inoperability.

A83
A. False
B. True
C. False
D. False
E. False

Carcinoma of the stomach is one of the cancers that can cause this mechanical haemolytic anaemia.

A84
A. True
B. False
C. True
D. False
E. False

Achalasia is a motility abnormality in the oesophagus characterised by aperistalsis. There are other causes of aperistalsis, such as oesophageal cancer. It is thought that dysphagia is more for liquids than solids, but this is an unreliable feature. A bird's beak deformity on barium meal is quite characteristic. A normal upper GI endoscopy suggests a motility abnormality but not necessarily achalasia. Stenosis of the lower oesophagus is not a feature in achalasia.

A85
A. True
B. True
C. True
D. True
E. True

Caffeine and GTN are known to relax the smooth muscle at the gastro-oesophageal junction. *H. pylori* eradication exacerbates gastro-oesophageal reflux by an undetermined mechanism. Previous partial gastrectomy and Billroth I reconstruction causes bile reflux. Stenting a benign or malignant lower oesophageal stricture maintains non-functional patency of the gastro-oesophageal junction.

A86
A. True
B. True
C. True
D. True
E. False

Resectability of cancer of the intra-thoracic oesophagus depends on the general condition of the patient and the stage of the disease determined by local infiltration and distant metastasis. The length of cancer is thought to correlate with its width and consequently local infiltration. Previous radiotherapy to the chest may make the operation more difficult but is not a contra-indication to resection.

A87
A. False
B. True
C. False
D. False
E. False

In 1724 Hermann Boerhaave described a fatal case of oesophageal perforation induced by severe retching. In classic Boerhaave's syndrome, acute gastric distress results in forceful vomiting, severe chest pain, collapse and hypotension from a complete tear of the lower oesophagus just above the cardia. Surgical management is influenced by the site of the perforation, the extent of the injury, the presence of co-existing oesophageal disease and the duration of the perforation, which determine the degree of mediastinitis. Mediastinitis is usually polymicrobial, caused by aerobes, anaerobes and fungal organisms. The diagnosis and post-operative checks are confirmed by a water-soluble contrast medium. Nasogastric intubation is best left until surgical management is undertaken, which should be urgent after the diagnosis is made. In selected cases conservative management may be appropriate and include multiple-suction drainage, but this is not the usual initial management.

A88
A. True
B. True
C. True
D. True
E. True

All the above conditions are recognised in causing non-cardiac chest pain. Diffuse oesophageal spasm (DOS) and high amplitude peristaltic contractions (nutcracker oesophagus) are primary motility abnormalities of the oesophagus. In DOS, less than 90% of the contractions are peristaltic. The condition can be a primary disorder or secondary to gastro-oesophageal reflux. Nutcracker oesophagus is characterised by peristaltic contractions with an amplitude of more than 140 mmHg. The condition commonly affects young females and manifests as chest pain. Gastro-oesophageal reflux with or without oesophagitis causes non-cardiac chest pain as a separate entity to heartburn.

A89
A. False
B. True
C. True
D. False
E. False

In 24-hour ambulatory oesophageal pH recordings, the pH probe is positioned 5 cm above the lower oesophageal high-pressure zone, determined manometrically. By convention a drop in pH below 4 defines a reflux event. The duration of reflux events and the longest reflux event defines the natural ability of the oesophagus to clear the refluxate either by neutralisation or by contractile expulsion from the oesophagus. Duodeno-gastric reflux, bile reflux or alkaline reflux cannot be determined by this method. Bilirubin or bile acid measurements are designed for this purpose (e.g. the Bilitec probe). The complete absence of reflux episodes in a 24-hour recording is unusual, but has several explanations such as the use of proton-pump inhibitors or malfunction of the probe, and rarely, the presence of a peptic stricture.

A90
A. False
B. False
C. False
D. True
E. True

Barrett's metaplasia in the lower oesophagus develops in 12–18% of patients with chronic gastro-oesophageal reflux disease. The condition is more common in white males who are smokers and it increases with age. The natural history of Barrett's metaplasia is similar to that of reflux oesophagitis that precedes it, in that it can undergo regression, stabilisation or progression. There is no evidence that the condition disappears by either medical or surgical therapy in patients with reflux. It is thought that gastro-oesophageal reflux leads to cardiac (gastric) metaplasia of the squamous epithelium in the lower oesophagus. Continued reflux into this region leads to intestinal metaplasia and consequently dysplasia. Although complications such as stricture, ulcer and dysplasia are more commonly associated with longer lengths of Barrett's change, patients with short-segment Barrett's mucosa are still considered to have a pre-malignant condition.

A91
A. False
B. False
C. True
D. False
E. True

The standard treatment for operable fit patients is oesophagectomy with lymphadenectomy. A combined approach of neo-adjuvant chemoradiation followed by radical surgery is appropriate for individual clinical use. Pre-operative radiotherapy alone contributes to lowering the incidence of local recurrence, but does not improve resectability or long-term survival, and hence is not recommended. Post-operative radiotherapy after a curative R0 resection is also not recommended since no survival benefit could be demonstrated. Post-operative radiotherapy after palliative resection (R1, R2) showed a reduction of local relapse and tracheobronchial obstruction, but with significant morbidity and mortality without a survival benefit. Although the presence of a tracheobronchial fistula is no longer considered an absolute contra-indication to radiotherapy, the use of radiotherapy in this group of patients is not recommended owing to the significant early complication rate. Radiotherapy to decrease pain from bone metastases is appropriate.

A92
A. False
B. True
C. False
D. False
E. True

Cisapride and metoclopramide are prokinetic agents. Sucralfate is a gastric and duodenal mucosal protective agent. Ranitidine is an H_2-receptor blocker which suppresses gastric acid output. Omeprazole is a proton-pump inhibitor that suppresses gastric acid output. The only drugs that are of established benefit in healing oesophagitis are those that achieve adequate acid suppression. Other drugs mentioned in the list can, in addition to acid suppression, improve the oesophagitis healing rates.

A93
A. False
B. True
C. True
D. True
E. True

Oesophageal diverticula are rare (in contrast to pharyngo-oesophageal diverticula). The congenital variety is very rare and may represent a remnant or forme fruste of a congenital tracheo-oesophageal fistula. Most oesophageal diverticula are thought to be pulsion diverticula. Oesophageal diverticula can given rise to dysphagia, chest pain or regurgitation. Excision of an oesophageal diverticulum is indicated if it is large enough to cause significant mechanical disturbance. Prior to diverticulectomy, a full pre-operative diagnosis must include demonstration of the diverticulum and the cause of it.

A94
A. False
B. True
C. True
D. False
E. True

The earliest and most subtle histological change in coeliac disease is an increase in intra-epithelial lymphocyte count on mucosal biopsy of the duodenum and jejunum. There is a strong genetic component through HLA association (DQw2) and family studies have shown that 10–20% of relatives may be affected. The anti-gliadin and anti-endomysial antibodies are useful in screening for coeliac disease, particularly in younger patients. Patients with coeliac disease may have an increased risk of oesophageal carcinoma as well as from small bowel lymphoma. In addition, there is an association between coeliac disease and insulin-dependent diabetes mellitus, and glucose malabsorption may contribute to difficulty in diabetic control in these individuals.

A95
A. False
B. True
C. True
D. True
E. False

DU is associated with acid hypersecretion. *H. pylori* infection remains the commonest cause, while Crohn's disease remains a rare cause. DU remains a common cause of upper GI haemorrhage.

A96
A. False
B. True
C. False
D. False
E. True

PPIs are non-competitive inhibitors of the proton pump, which have greater pH-raising efficacy in *H. pylori*-infected subjects. They reduce the accuracy of urease-dependent tests, such as the CLO and urea breath test. Most gastric ulcers remain *H. pylori* related and, therefore, *H. pylori* eradication remains the most important treatment for them.

A97
A. False
B. True
C. True
D. False
E. False

H. pylori-related gastric ulcers remain the most common type and are associated with low or normal acid secretion. The majority are benign, although endoscopic biopsies to exclude malignancy pre- and post-therapy remain the norm. Duodenal ulcers remain the most prevalent form of PU and most common cause of upper GI bleeding.

A98
A. False
B. False
C. True
D. False
E. False

The ECL cell is stimulated by gastrin, acting at gastrin receptors to cause release of histamine, its main vesicular constituent. This then acts at H_2-receptors on parietal cells to stimulate acid secretion. The ECL cell is the cell type from which gastric carcinoids arise.

A99
A. True
B. True
C. False
D. True
E. False

Populations with high dietary salt and achlorhydria have been associated with distal gastric carcinoma. Coeliac disease has been associated with oesophageal and small bowel carcinoma. Duodenal ulcer patients have a lower risk of gastric carcinoma than the rest of the population.

A100
A. False
B. True
C. True
D. True
E. True

H. pylori is commonly associated with the more common distal gastric cancer, causing atrophic gastritis, with consequent achlorhydria and bacterial overgrowth. The incidence is higher in countries such as Chile and Japan, probably reflecting environmental factors. Incidences of proximal cancer are increasing in Western countries.

A101
A. True
B. False
C. True
D. False
E. True

Among the non-NSAID causes of *H. pylori*-negative duodenal ulcer disease to be considered are Crohn's coeliac and hyperparathyroidism. Schistosomiasis and ACE inhibitors have no known association.

A102
A. True
B. False
C. False
D. False
E. True

Portal hypertensive gastropathy is by definition caused by portal hypertension. Watermelon stomach is the name given to the characteristic appearance in the antrum of the stomach that is often but not always caused by portal hypertension. These appearances have been described in autoimmune diseases, connective tissue disorders and pernicious anaemia in the absence of portal hypertension. Hereditary haemorrhagic telangiectasia can be a cause of cirrhosis and, therefore, portal hypertension, but the reverse is not true.

A103
A. False
B. False
C. True
D. False
E. False

Most iron absorption occurs in the duodenum and proximal small intestine. Gastric acid allows iron taken in the diet to become soluble and, therefore, available for absorption. Patients with achlorhydria, e.g. following partial gastrectomy or on acid-suppressing drugs, will have impaired iron absorption. Polyphenols found in tea are potent inhibitors of iron absorption, whereas vitamin C enhances iron absorption by helping keep iron in a soluble form. There is no mechanism for iron excretion in humans.

A104
A. False
B. True
C. False
D. True
E. False

Bleeding from oesophageal varices is more likely if the varices are large, red spots or weals are present on the varices, if the patient has a bacterial infection and if the patient's liver disease is graded as Child-Pugh C. If liver disease is due to alcohol, abstinence can make the varices regress or even disappear. Bleeding from varices does not occur unless the hepatic venous pressure gradient (the difference in pressure between the hepatic vein and portal vein) is greater than 10–12 mmHg.

A105
A. True
B. False
C. True
D. False
E. False

Non-selective β-blockers, such as propranolol, reduce portal pressure by reducing the flow of blood into the portal circulation. This is achieved by a reduction in cardiac output (β_1-adrenoreceptor blockade) and splanchnic vasoconstriction (β_2-adrenoreceptor blockade). Cardioselective β-blockers, such as atenolol, do reduce portal pressure but the effect is not as great as non-selective β-blockers as they do not cause splanchnic vasoconstriction. Therefore they are not used. Glypressin is an intravenous drug used for acute variceal bleeding and not for prophylaxis. Nitrates lower portal pressure by reducing the resistance to portal collateral blood flow and causing reflex splanchnic vasoconstriction in response to reduced arterial pressures.

A106
A. True
B. True
C. True
D. True
E. False

Partial gastrectomy causes, and pernicious anaemia is associated with, achlorhydria. Gastric acid is important for allowing non-haem iron to become soluble and available for absorption. Haem iron (i.e. iron from haemoglobin or myoglobin) is more readily absorbed and is less influenced by gastric acid and other food components than non-haem iron. In industrialised countries haem iron composes 10–15% of ingested iron, but about one-third of absorbed iron.

A107
A. False
B. False
C. True
D. True
E. False

H. pylori amoxycillin resistance is virtually unknown. Although resistance to other antibiotics may contribute to treatment failure, compliance, often due to common side-effects with treatment, is more important. At present *H. pylori* eradication therapy is only recommended for peptic ulcer and gastric lymphoma.

A108
A. True
B. False
C. True
D. True
E. True

The biopsy urease test depends on the production by *H. pylori* of an enzyme (urease) that digests urea to carbon dioxide and ammonia. This results in a net production of alkali that changes the colour of the pH indicator phenol red from yellow to red, indicating a positive result. A decrease in the number of bacteria or their migration to the proximal stomach will interfere with the test. *Proteus* spp. also produce the urease enzyme and can thus give a false positive.

A109
A. False
B. False
C. False
D. False
E. False

Mallory–Weiss tear is a mucosal tear occurring at the oesophago-gastric junction. It usually resolves spontaneously with no long-term sequelae. Occasionally treatment is required to arrest haemorrhage (medical, endoscopic or surgery).

A110
A. False
B. True
C. False
D. True
E. False

Two types of carcinoma of the oesophagus are identified. Squamous carcinoma is the most common type world-wide and is associated with many risk factors which are predominantly causes of physical, chemical or biological irritation to the lining of the oesophagus. Adenocarcinoma arises in association with Barrett's oesophagus. surgical resection is the treatment of choice as it offers a chance of cure if the lesion is identified early. Palliation for dysphagia is best achieved by the deployment of a self-expanding stent, either endoscopically or radiologically, with additional chemotherapy and/or radiotherapy, depending on the patient's clinical status. Barium radiology may occasionally be misleading, and endoscopy with biopsy and cytology is the investigation of choice.

A111
A. True
B. False
C. False
D. False
E. True

Oesophageal motility disorders may present with chest pain or dysphagia. Diffuse oesophageal spasm may be seen occasionally on endoscopy as coil-like spasms. The barium swallow appearance of these spasms is known as a 'corkscrew' oesophagus. 'Nutcracker' oesophagus refers to hypertensive normally propagated peristalsis. Calcium antagonists may be useful in treatment, but not β-blockers.

Achalasia of the cardia is treated by balloon dilatation of the oesophagus. Botulinum toxin injections locally are also effective. Metal stents are deployed only as palliation for oesophageal carcinoma.

A112
A. False
B. False
C. True
D. True
E. False

Branch-chain amino acids as a group include valine, leucine and isoleucine. Phenylalaline and tyrosine are aromatic amino acids. It was suggested that an infusion of branch-chain amino acids is effective treatment of hepatic encephalopathy. This has not been proven but it has been demonstrated that fusions of branch-chain amino acids improves nitrogen balance in chronic liver disease. They are found in high concentrations of muscle and are utilised as a source of amino acids in patients with chronic liver disease, hence the muscle wasting.

A113
A. False
B. True
C. True
D. False
E. False

Active ATPhase hydrogen pumps are found only in parietal cells and renal tubular cells, but proton-pump-inhibitor drugs are ineffective on renal tubules owing to differences in intracellular pH.

A114
A. True
B. False
C. False
D. False
E. True

There is a well-established increased risk in tuberculosis following gastric surgery owing to the loss of acid following surgery which is known to inhibit the growth of bacteria. Folic acid malabsorption is normal following gastric surgery but there is a loss of B_{12} owing to a loss of intrinsic factor, and hence a megaloblastic anaemia is common, being associated with B_{12} deficiency. Surgery controls, but does not always eradicate, *H. pylori*. This organism in the gastric remnant may well account for the increased risk of gastric malignancy in the operated stomach.

A115
A. True
B. False
C. False
D. False
E. True

Total parenteral nutrition can cause cholestatic jaundice and, therefore, patients on TPN should have regular 'liver function' tests. Recent studies have shown that this is tolerated for short periods when given through a peripheral line. There is no evidence of its use in short-bowel syndrome. Enteral feeding would be the treatment of choice, nor does it cause pancreatitis or diarrhoea.

A116
A. True
B. False
C. True
D. True
E. False

It has been clearly demonstrated that patients who are refed may develop the refeeding syndrome, which is associated with an increase in metabolic rate, and causes a fall in most electrolytes including calcium and potassium. As a consequence of change in electrolyte status, patients may have cardiac and respiratory failure precipitated. In addition, especially with the early introduction of carbohydrate, Wernicke's encephalopathy may occur.

A117
A. False
B. True
C. True
D. False
E. False

Achalasia is rare under the age of 15 and is more likely to be found in the older age group. Owing to the oesophagus's failure to empty, there is spillage during sleep of oesophageal content into the trachea, causing coughing. There is a known risk of oesophageal cancer with achalasia. Dysphagia is a far more common presentation symptom in the elderly. Treatment with cisapride would not be very effective.

A118
A. False
B. True
C. True
D. False
E. True

A119
A. False
B. True
C. True
D. True
E. True

Although commonly associated with the pancreas, tumours causing Zollinger-Ellison syndrome have also been well documented as occurring in the duodenal wall, ovary and parathyroid gland.

A120
A. True
B. True
C. False
D. True
E. True

A number of drugs, including slow-release potassium chloride preparations, tetracycline and doxycycline, have been shown to cause oesophageal ulceration, particularly in the elderly. Anti-cholinergic agents slow gastric emptying, reduce lower oesophageal sphincter pressure and reduce the volume and alkalinity of saliva, all of which contribute to gastro-oesophageal reflux. NSAIDs can produce ulcers at almost any site in the gastrointestinal tract, but in the stomach these are characteristically prepyloric. The use of suppositories does not prevent the formation of prepyloric ulcers. Mefenamic acid may cause inflammation of the terminal ileum with subsequent malabsorption. NSAIDs may give rise to circumferential ulceration in the gastric antrum, small or large intestine, and this may be replaced by fibrous tissue forming a diaphragm across the lumen of the bowel, causing obstruction.

A121
A. True
B. False
C. True
D. True
E. False

Drugs, such as anti-malarials, oral contraceptives and phenothiazines, may cause oral pigmentation while tetracycline ingestion in children during tooth formation may cause staining/pigmentation of the teeth. There is no specific reason why oral pigmentation should occur in ulcerative colitis. Diffuse pigmentation of the buccal mucosa may be seen in Addison's disease. ACTH-producing bronchogenic carcinomas may present with oral pigmentation, and if pigmentation is localised, malignant melanoma must be excluded. Chronic laxative abuse can give rise to pigmentation in the large intestine.

A122
A. False
B. True
C. True
D. True
E. True

Crohn's disease can classically affect any part of the gastrointestinal tract from the mouth to the anus, while oral manifestations of ulcerative colitis are more rare and include pyoderma gangrenosum, recurrent aphthous stomatitis and pyostomatitis vegetans. Remodelling of facial bones occurs in the haemoglobinopathies owing to the expansion of the marrow cavity. A number of oral manifestations of cystic fibrosis may be seen in addition to submandibular salivary gland enlargement, including hypoplastic teeth. Amyloidosis may cause macroglossia in myelomatosis.

A123
A. False
B. True
C. True
D. True
E. False

Carcinoma of the oesophagus appears to be a disease of poverty and malnutrition. The quantity and type of alcohol consumed or tobacco smoked appears to be important in the development of oesophageal cancer in some areas. There is a reported 22-fold increased risk of development of oesophageal cancer in patients with corrosive oesophageal strictures. Gastro-oesophageal reflux is associated with the development of adenocarcinoma of the oesophagus and there is little evidence that it is associated with an increased risk of squamous carcinoma.

A124
A. False
B. True
C. True
D. False
E. False

Gastric secretion from gastric glands is about 2500 ml/day. Energy for pumping H^+ out of the parietal cells is appreciable and provided by hydrolysis of ATP. High secretion of H^+ during a meal can cause high pH in the blood and thus alkaline urine in the post-prandial tide. Regulation of H^+–K^+ ATPase is via intracellular protein kinases which are switched on via acetyl choline and gastrin. These raise intracellular Ca^{++} and histamine which increases intracellular cyclic AMP. Prostaglandin E series inhibit gastric secretion, which partly explains the increased incidences of ulcers in patients taking anti-inflammatory drugs that inhibit prostaglandin synthesis through inhibition of cyclo-oxygenase enzymes.

A125
A. True
B. True
C. False
D. False
E. True

IF is a MW 45 000 glycoprotein secreted in the body of the stomach by the parietal cells. It becomes firmly bound to cyanocobalamin in the intestine. The complex binds to specific receptors in the ileum and the cyanocobalamin is transferred across the intestinal epithelium, possibly by endocytosis. The exact details of this are uncertain for this large complex molecule to be absorbed. Trypsin is required for the process to be efficient and absorption of cyanocobalamin is sometimes decreased in patients with pancreatic insufficiency. Patients with total gastrectomy and patients with atrophic gastritis and achlorhydria need parenteral cyanocobalamin to bypass the deficiency of the IF.

A126
A. True
B. False
C. True
D. False
E. False

About 1500 ml of saliva are secreted per day. The resting pH of the gland is 7.0; active secretion is pH 8.0. The gland secretes two digestive enzymes – lingual lipase on the tongue and ptyalin (salivary amylase) from the glands. The sub-mandibular glands provide 70% of the secreted volume of a moderate viscous secretion. The secretion at rest is hypotonic for all glands but in high secretion rates it becomes almost isotonic. The control of salivary secretion is neural via the parasympathetic systems, producing a watery saliva with low organic content. There is a pronounced vasodilatation of the gland owing to the local release of VIP. Food in the mouth causes reflex stimulation to vagal efferents at the lower end of the oesophagus. In humans, sight, smell, and even the thought of food, makes the mouth water. Secretion is reduced by atropine and other cholinergic blocking agents. Stimulation of the sympathetic nervous system causes vasoconstriction and secretions of small amounts of saliva rich in organic constituents from the sub-mandibular gland.

A127
A. False
B. True
C. False
D. True
E. False

Receptors in the posterior fauces, the posterior tongue and the pharynx trigger impulses in the trigeminal, glossopharyngeal and vagus nerves to initiate swallowing. They are integrated in the nucleus of the tractus solitarius in the medulla oblongata. The efferent fibres pass to the pharyngeal muscles via trigeminal, facial and hypoglossal nerves. The voluntary action of collecting oral contents in a bolus on the tongue and then propelling them backwards in to the pharynx starts a wave of involuntary contraction, inhibiting respiration and closing the epiglottis via the pharyngeal muscles' raising of the larynx.

Normal voluntary swallowing frequently occurs while eating, but this swallowing also continues between meals. The total number of swallows per day is approximately 600: 200 while eating and drinking, and 350 while awake without food, and 50 while asleep.

At the pharyngo-oesophageal junction there is a 3 cm segment of oesophagus whose resting tension is high. This is known as the cricopharyngeus muscle. This relaxes reflexly upon swallowing, permitting swallowed material to enter the oesophagus. A peristalsis develops behind the bolus which sweeps it down the oesophagus at about 4 cm/s. In the upright position, food and fluid fall ahead of the peristaltic waves. The muscles of the gastro-oesophageal junction are also tonically active and relax ahead of the peristaltic wave. This relaxation may be mediated by neural secretion of nitrogen oxide (NO). The tonic activity helps to prevent reflux of gastric contents.